1

A Miracle at Bates Memorial

ISBN: 978-1-7328197-1-9

Copyright © 2018 Gin Noon Spaulding by

BFF Publishing House
PO Box 180234
Tallahassee, Florida 32318
Illustrator: Aranahaj Iqbal

For permission requests, to purchase this book in bulk or for special orders, write to the author, addressed "Attention: Permissions Coordinator," at:

theadventuresoflili2003@gmail.com

www.gustgin-author.com

BFF Publishing House is a Limited Liability Corporation dedicated wholly to the appreciation and publication of children and adults for the advancement of diversification in literature.

For more information on publishing contact

Antionette Mutcherson at

bff@bffpublishinghouse.com

Website: bffpublishinghouse.com

Published in the United States by

BFF Publishing House

Tallahassee, Florida First Edition, 2018

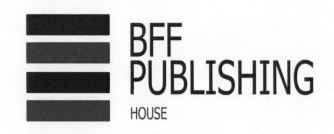

Dedication

Dedication

I'd like to dedicate my first book to my beautiful, loving mother, Lisa Renee Noon, who taught me that I could do ANYTHING I wanted to do and that I was just as good as ANYONE, if not better!

To my husband, Larry Spaulding, for supporting me through all of my big ideas, for just trusting God with me, and riding along being my Ride or Die partner for LIFE! Love you Lare Bear!

To my daughter, Maleah Antonia Spaulding. You are my inspiration. Without you, this book series would've never been written. You have taught me so much about myself and others, especially the children in my classroom. Thank you for being you. I'm so proud to be your mommy. I love you more than words could ever say!

Gin Noon- Spaulding

Dedication

I'd like to dedicate my first book to my beautiful, loving mother, Lisa Renee Noon, who taught me that I could do ANYTHING I wanted to do and that I was just as good as ANYONE, if not better!

To my husband, Larry Spaulding, for supporting me through all of my big ideas, for just trusting God with me, and riding along being my Ride or Die partner for LIFE! Love you Lare Bear!

To my daughter, Maleah Antonia Spaulding. You are my inspiration. Without you, this book series would've never been written. You have taught me so much about myself and others, especially the children in my classroom. Thank you for being you. I'm so proud to be your mommy. I love you more than words could ever say!

Gin Noon- Spaulding

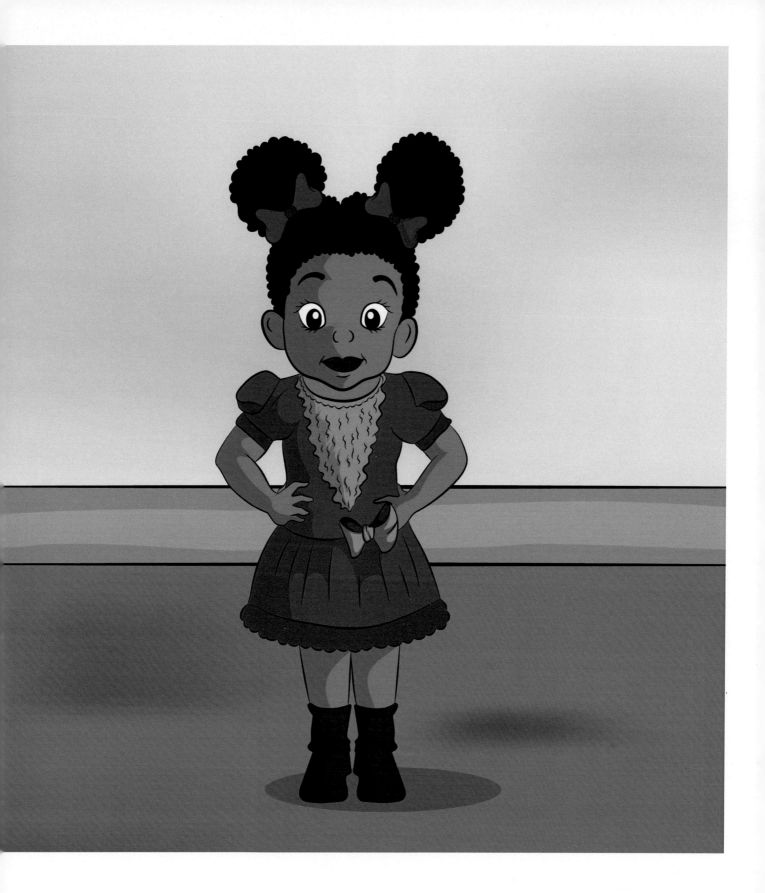

"Hi. My name is Maleah Antonia Spaulding, but most people call me Li-Li. My daddy made up that name just for me!"

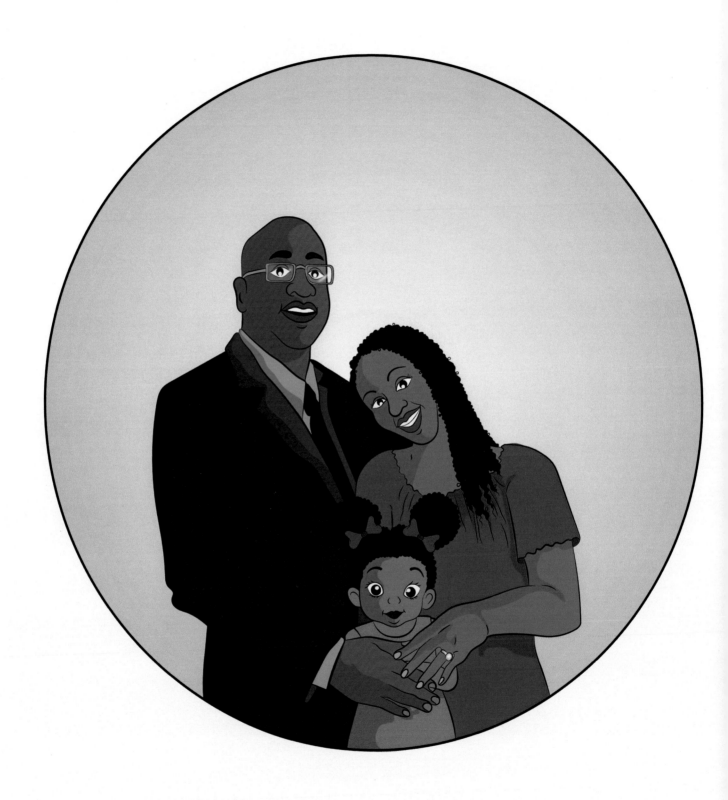

My name Maleah means
"Unique Little Girl/
Beautiful Young Woman," my mama says.
I just like to be called Li-Li.

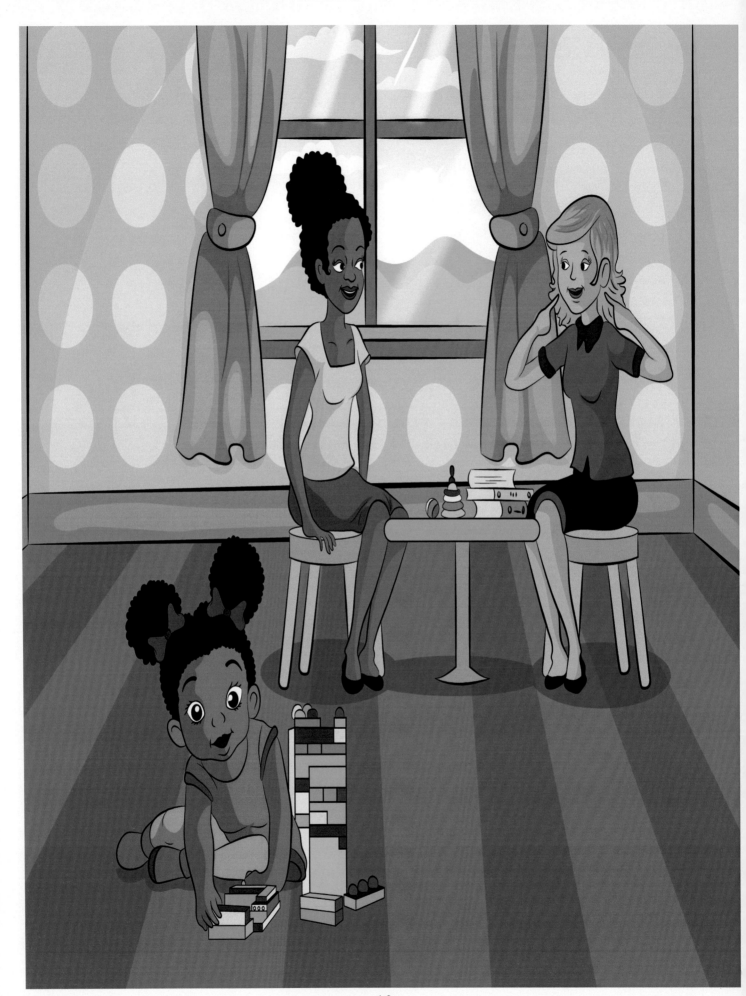

I heard my big friend tell my mama that I have a speech delay and sensory issues. I don't know what that means. All I know is that I like playing with my friend every week. We swing on a special swing from the ceiling, play games, do Brain Gym, jump on the trampoline, and have LOTS of fun.

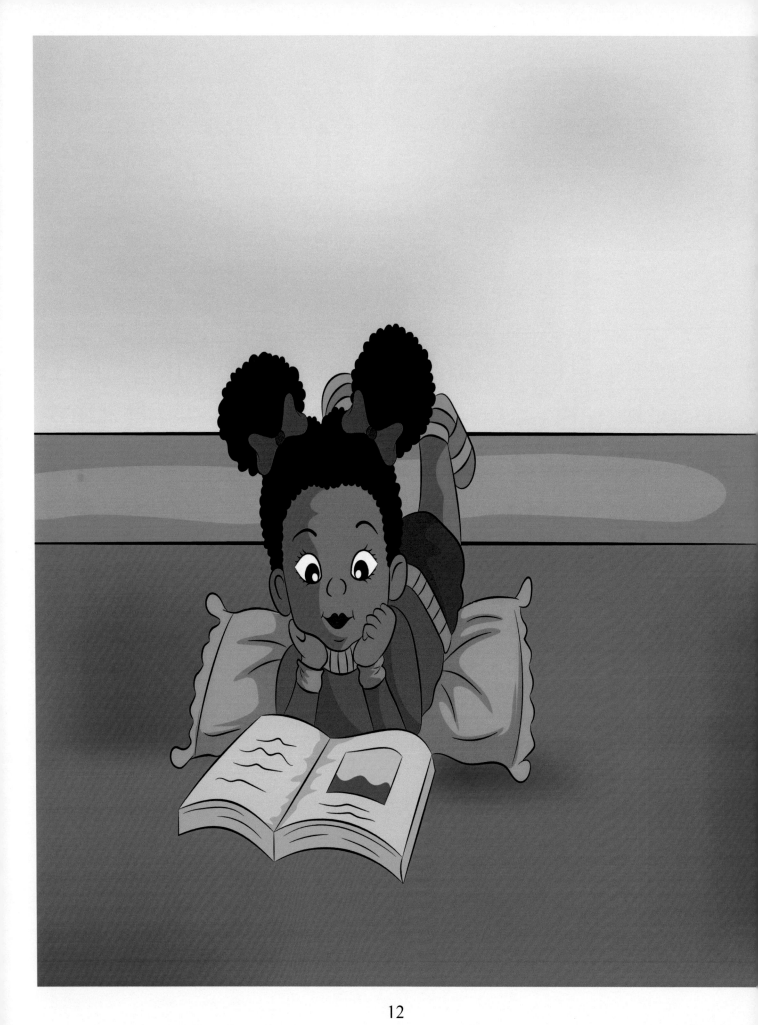

I LOVE so many things! Reading my books, listening to my mommy, daddy, or teacher read, counting to 100 and watching Baby Einstein are all my favorites.

I really LOOOOVVVVVEEE my church!

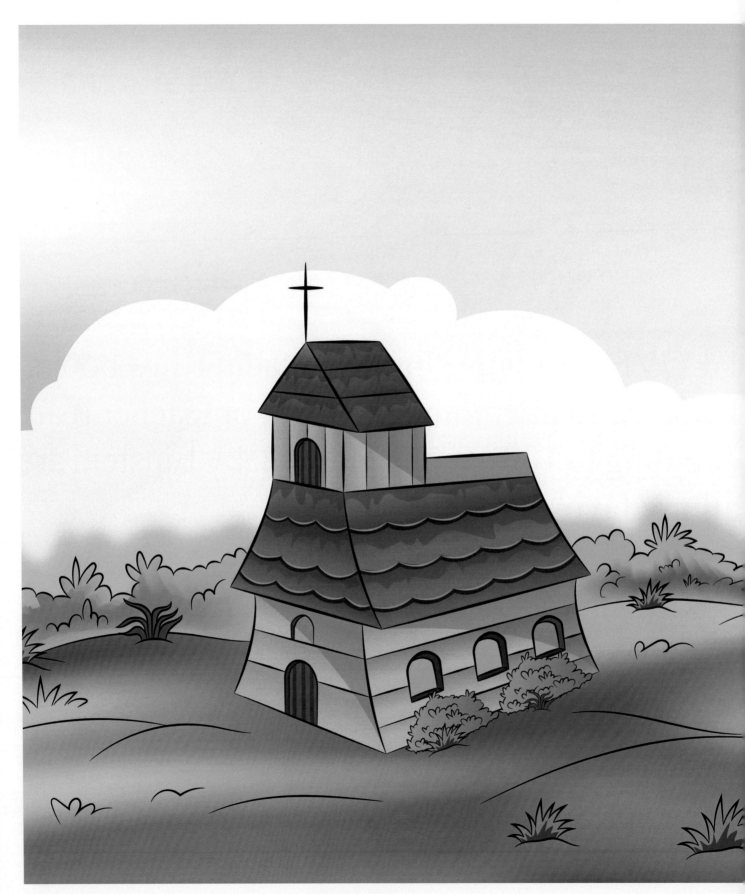

The choir sings soooo well. My favorite song is, "God Will Show Up and Show Out!"

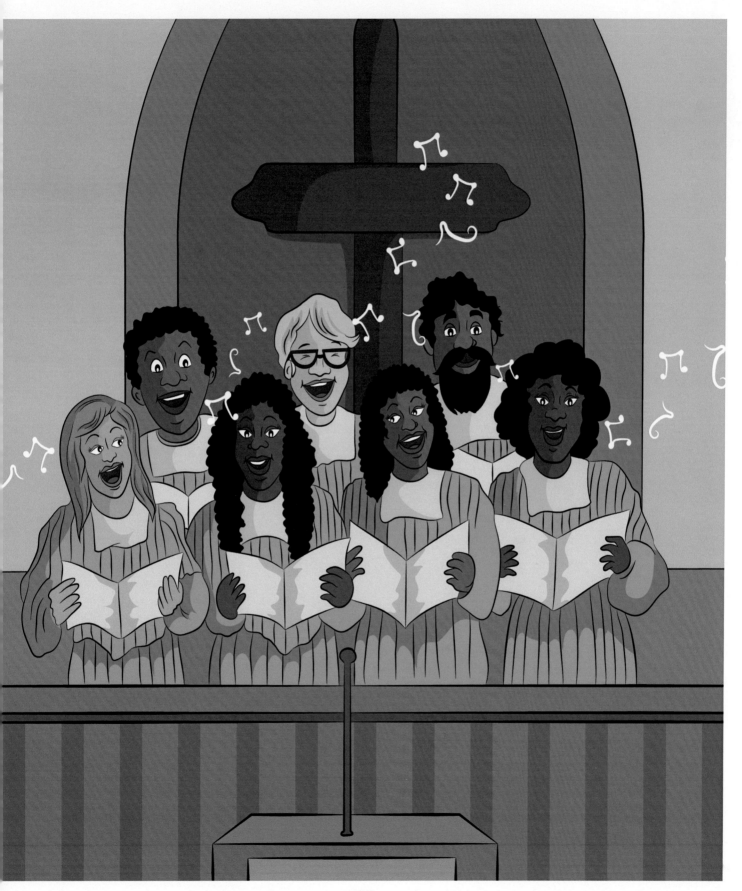

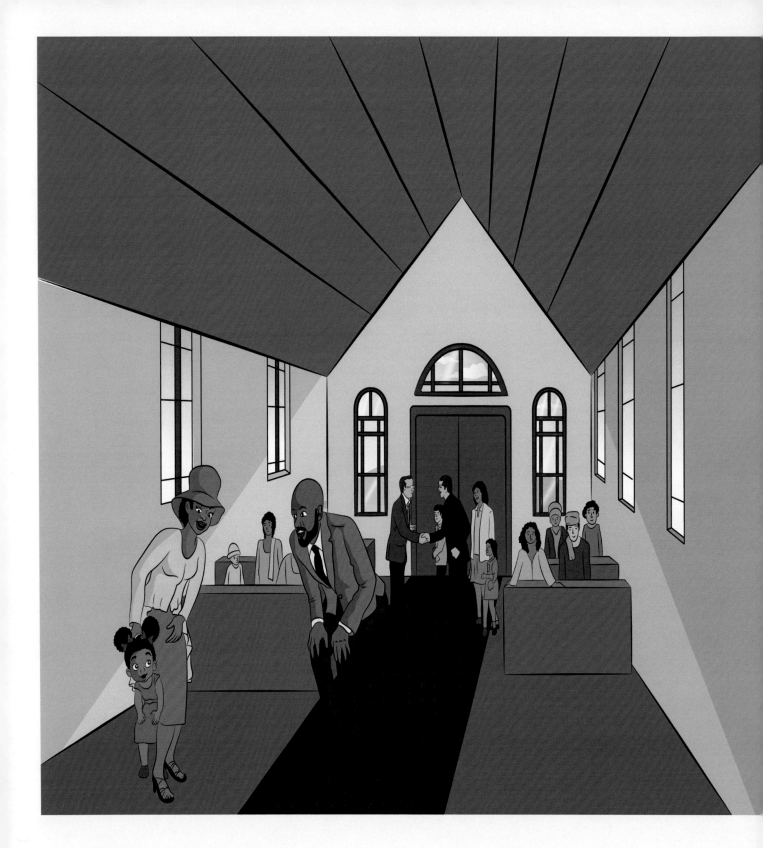

I LOOOVVVVVEEE my pastor. He always smiles and tries to talk to me. I hide behind my mama. I like him, but I don't want anyone looking at me. I look down. I want my pastor to know I really like him, but I don't want to look at him.

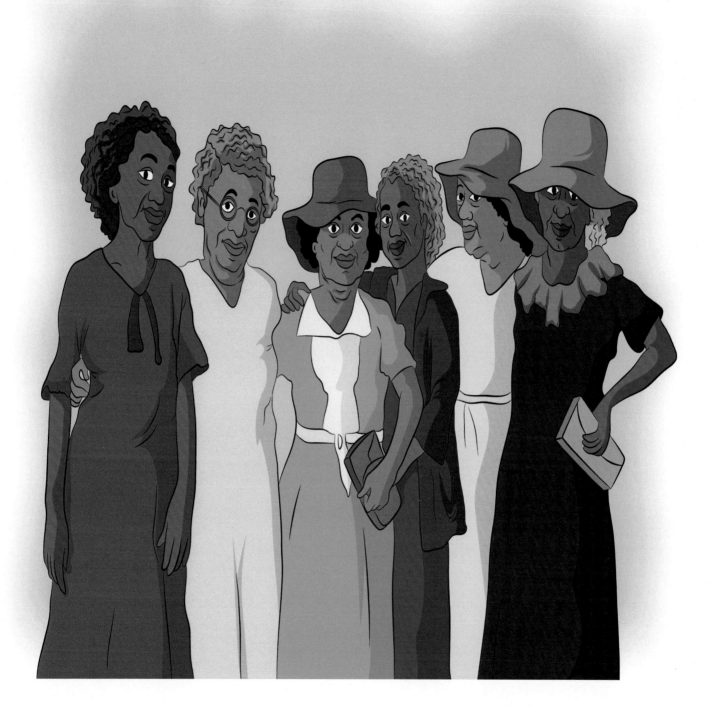

I LOOOOVVVVVEEE the nice, silver haired ladies. They give me candy when my mama's not looking. My mama says candy turns me into a wild thing... NOT! I just get a little excited with candy. What's wrong with that?

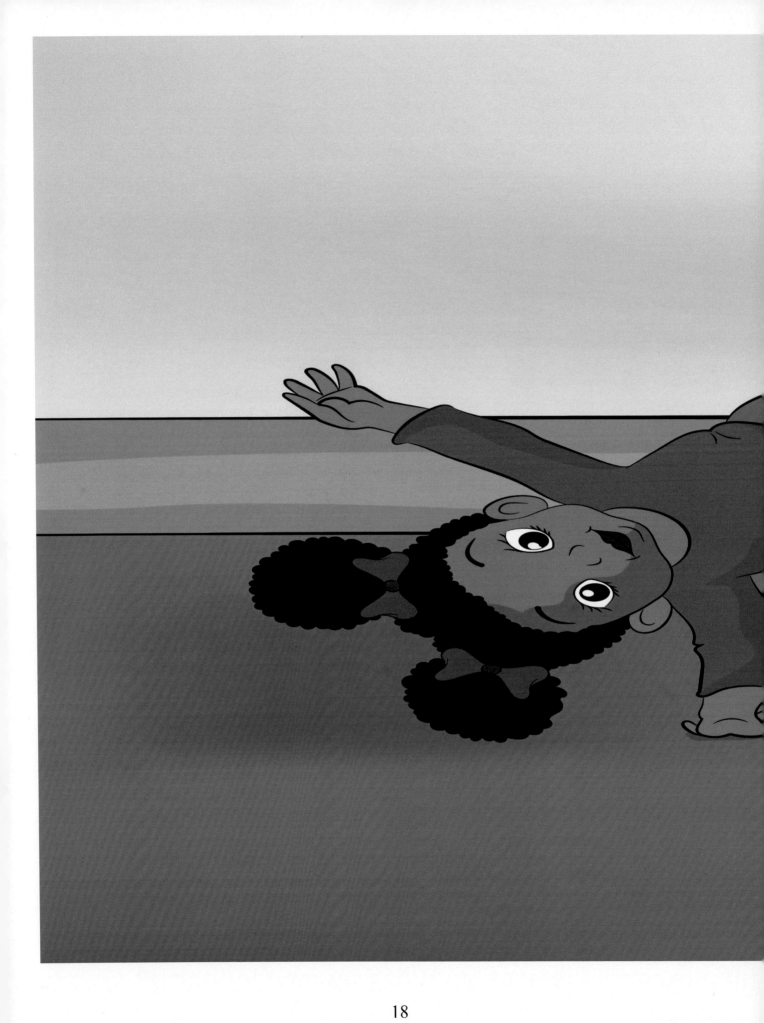

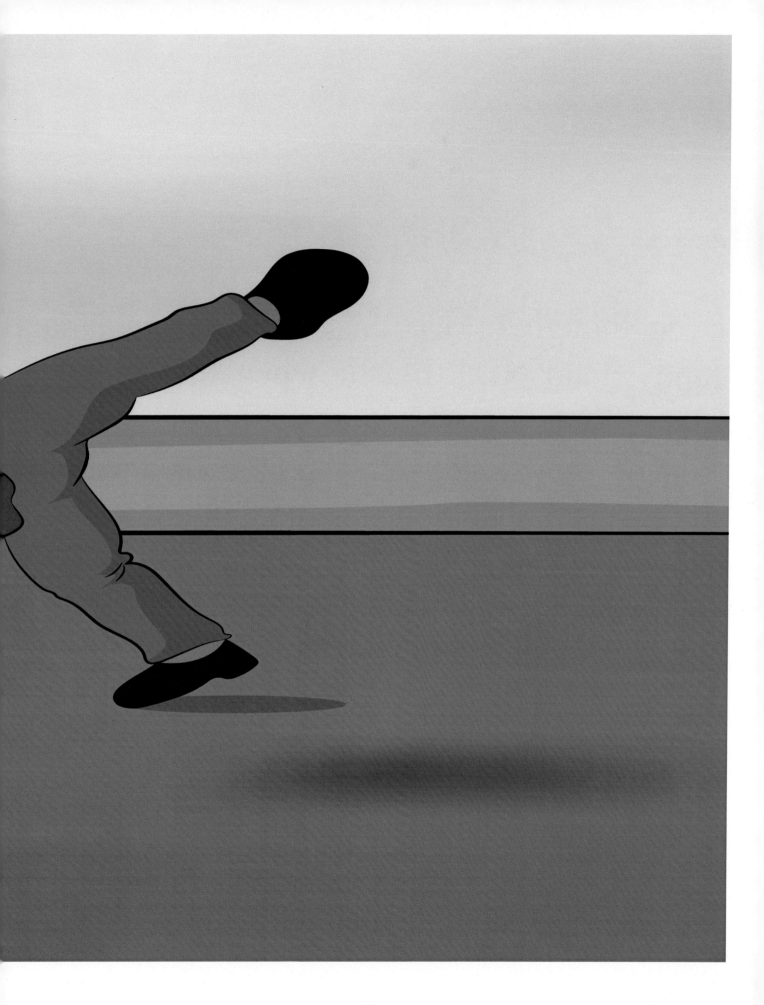

Even though I love the silver haired ladies' candy, I do NOT like it when they hug and squeeze me. I HATE it.

Don't they know it hurts me? I feel so smoothered, like I have a bunch of covers piled on my head and I just can't get them off. I can't breathe! I cry and say NOOOO! My mama always looks embarrassed and says, "Oh, Li-Li is just tired!"

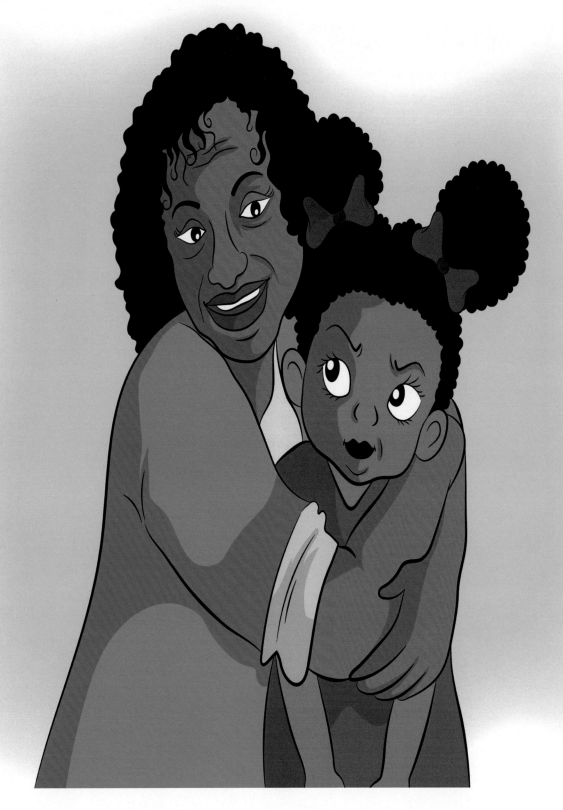

I want to say, "No I am NOT." I just don't want to be hugged and squeezed and NEVER kissed. NOOOO!!! All I can do is squirm, move, and try to get away.

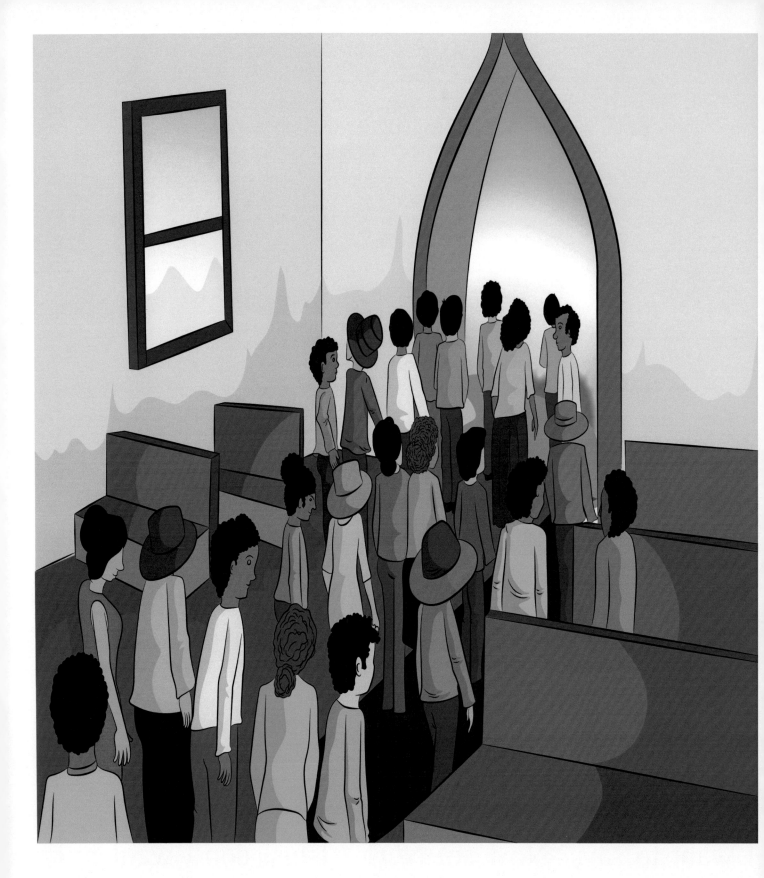

Do you wanna know what I hate the most? LEAVING MY CHURCH! My mommy always wants to go her way. It is too loud, too crowded, too noisy, and TOO MUCH!

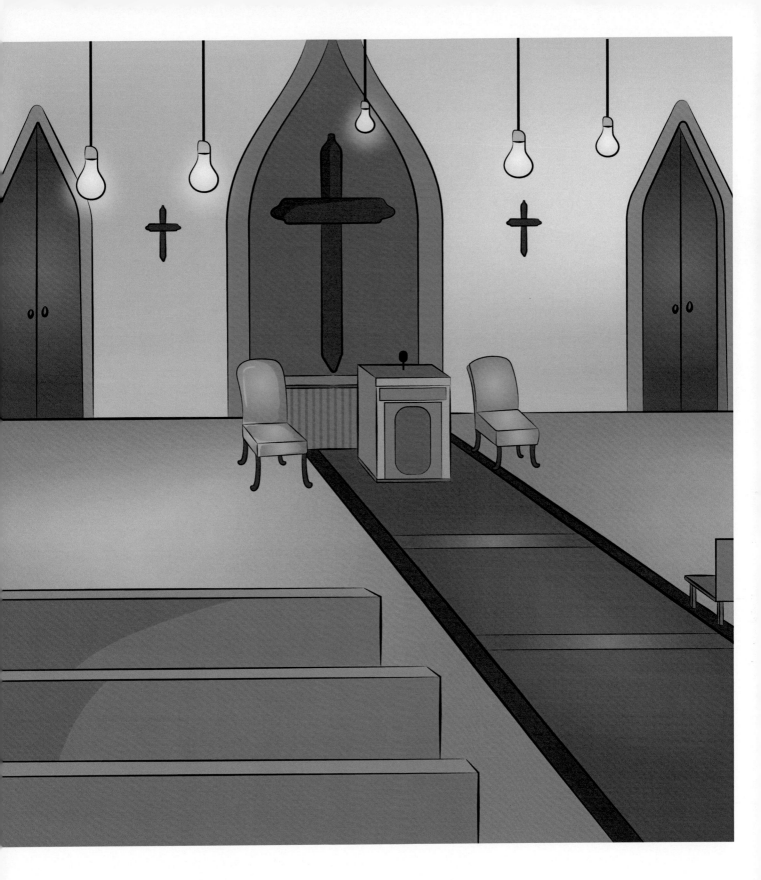

I always want to go my way where there is NO CROWD.
See, no people that way at all.

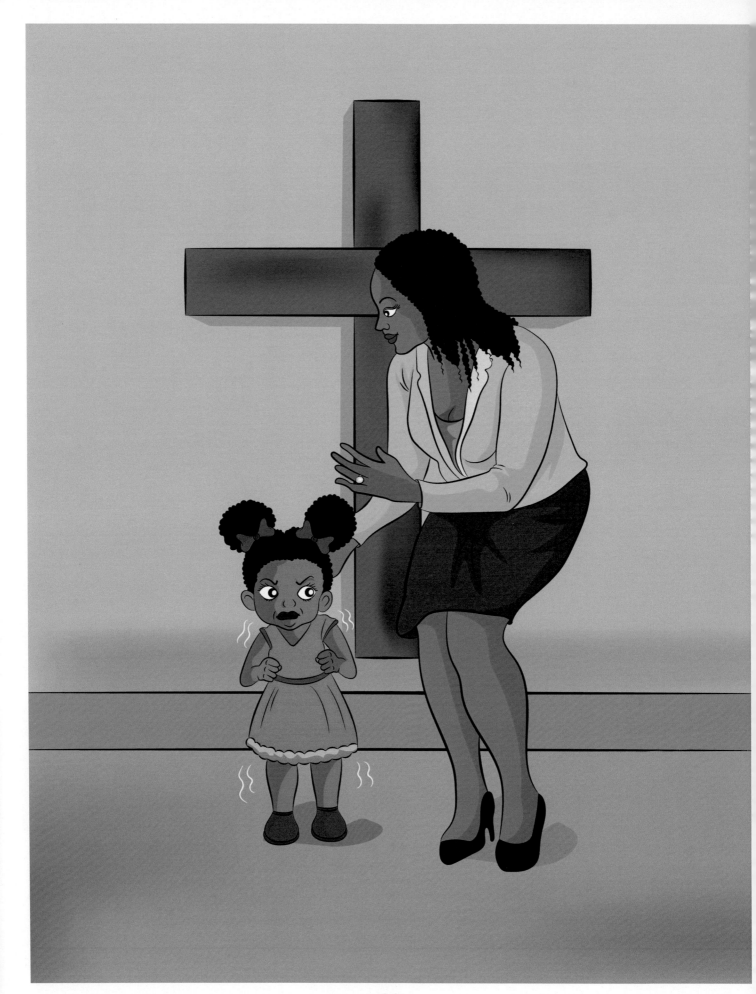

I try to tell my mommy that her way hurts me. All the people talking at one time makes my head hurt. It feels like pins pricking my skin, but all I can get out is, "Nooooo!"

My mama says, "Now Li-Li, Come on now. Let's get it together. This way is quicker. We can get to the car in no time!"

I want to say... "Mommy... please... it hurts me to go that way. It is too loud. The people bump into me. The lights are too bright. They hurt my eyes. I just can't!"

But, "Noooo, I wanna go this way!" is all that comes out.

I go boneless and begin to scream, cry, and shout... wishing my daddy wasn't Deaconing.

He would let me go my way. Then... a miracle happens. Just when I am ready to let it all hang out and have a...

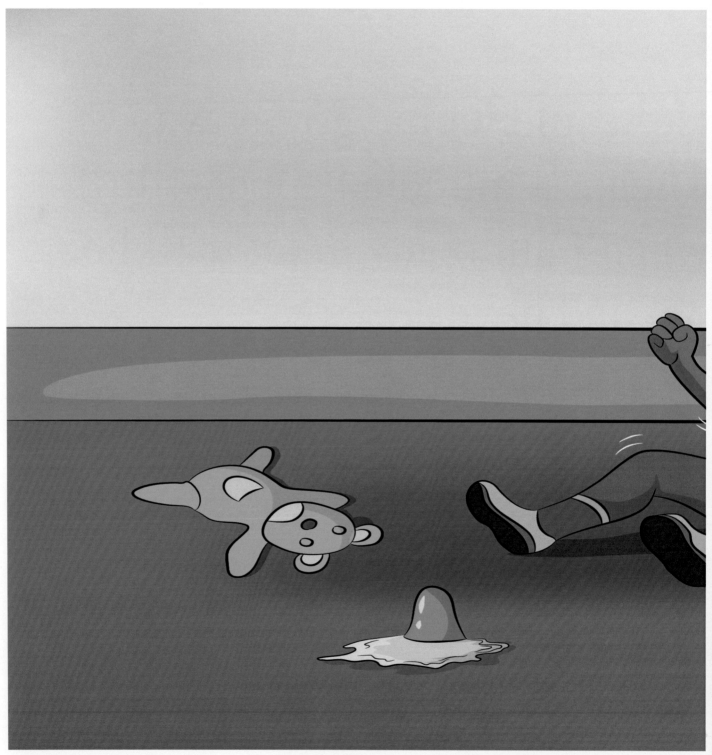

LETDOWN

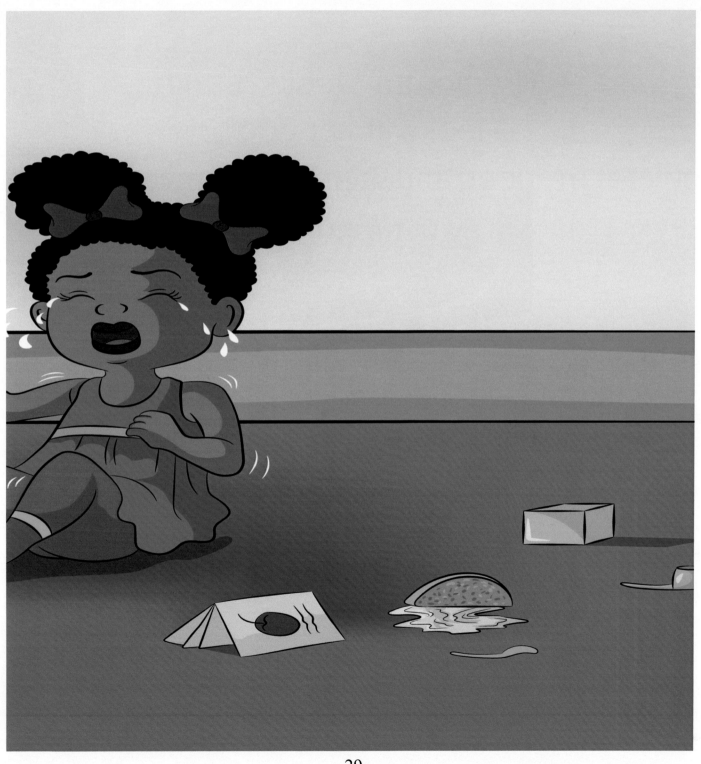

My mommy looks at me,
looks at her door,
looks at my door, and then back at me. Then, she
says, "Maleah, we are going to go your way."

It is a MIRACLE!

My mommy gets it!

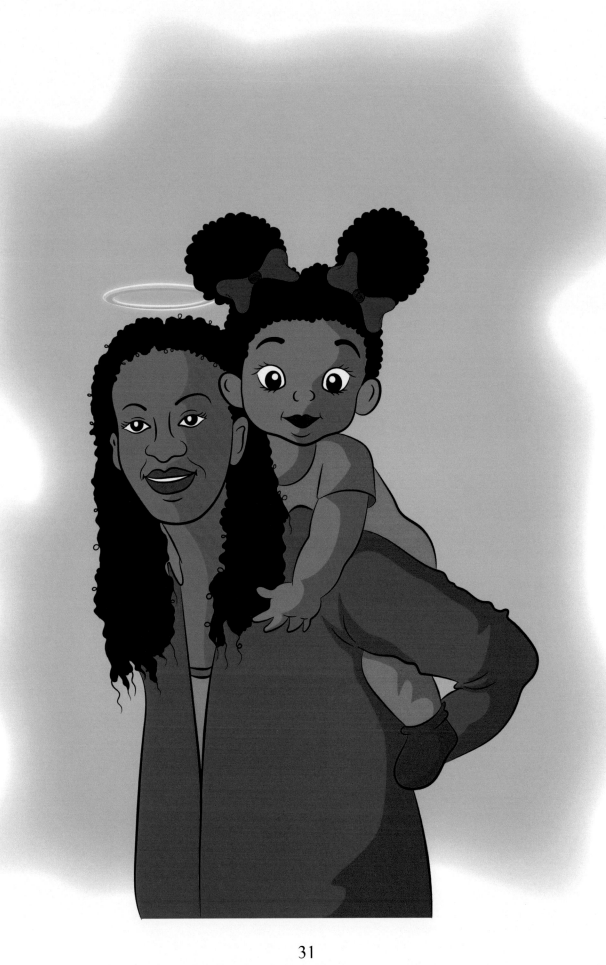

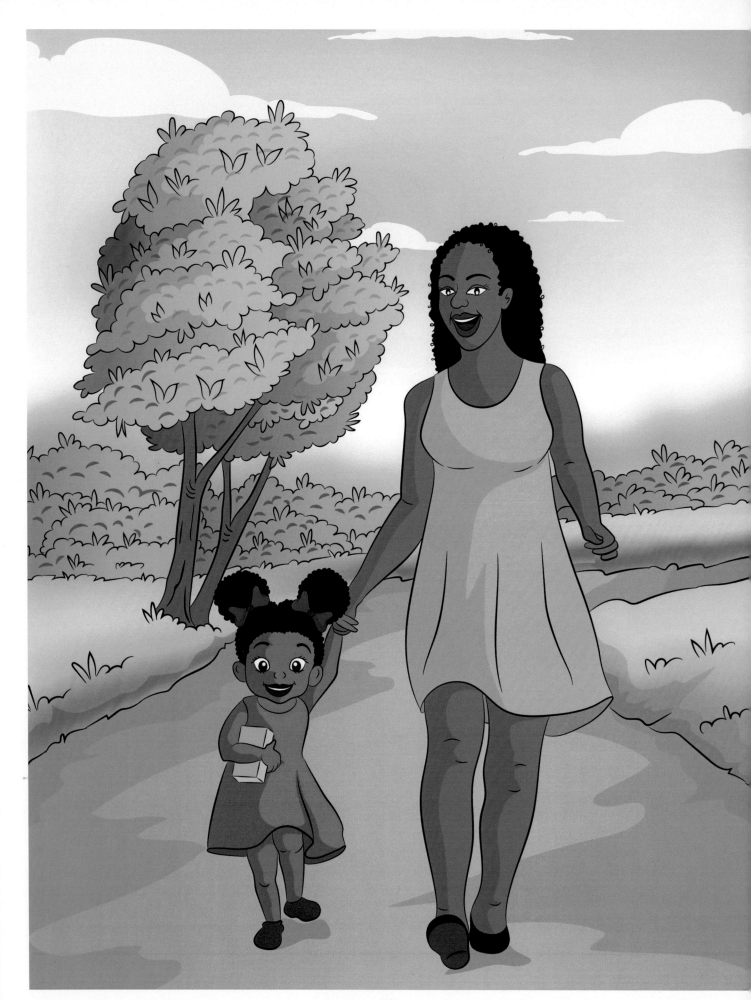

Right away,
I jump to my feet,
smile at my mommy, and say...
"Come on mommy!"

And that was the miracle at Bates Memorial.

The End

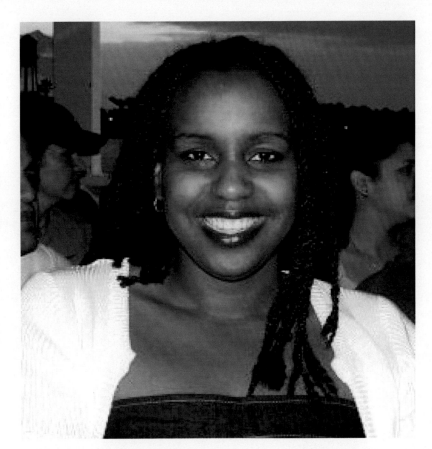

Mrs. Gin Noon-Spaulding has enjoyed writing since she was a young child, growing up in Tullahoma, Tennessee. She often has entertained friends and family with endless stories about life in a small town, funny tales of her parents' upbringing, and her own life experiences. Mrs. Spaulding holds a BS in Education from Austin Peay State University in Clarksville, TN and a Master of Education Degree from the University of Louisville.

Mrs. Spaulding lives in Louisville, KY with her husband of 17 years, Larry, and their wiz-kid daughter, Maleah, the star of The Adventures of Li-Li children's book series. Mrs. Spaulding is a recently retired teacher of 27 years from JCPS and plans to write even more stories, volunteer, and be the best wife, mother, friend, sister, daughter, and person she can possibly be.

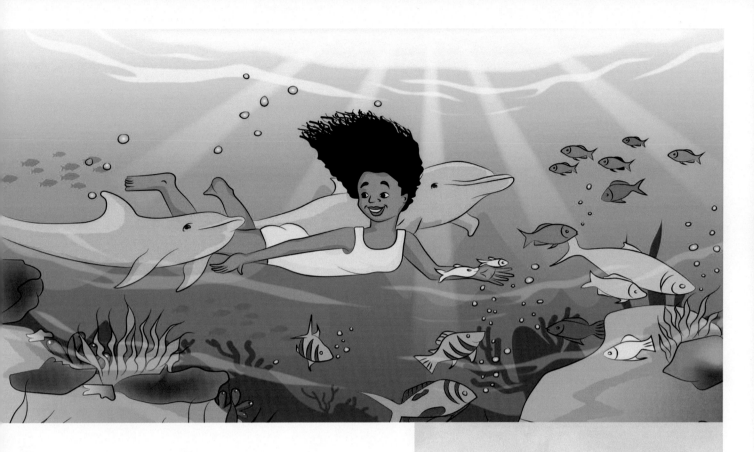

Aranahaj Iqbal has been an illustrator for more than five years. Illustrating children's books is her specialty! She especially enjoys working with book series and long term projects.

Please check out her portfolio work at the following places:
Facebook: www.facebook.com/aranahajart
Instagram: @aranahajiqbal
Twitter:
Aranahaji (ARANAHAHJI)
Website: www.aranahajart.com

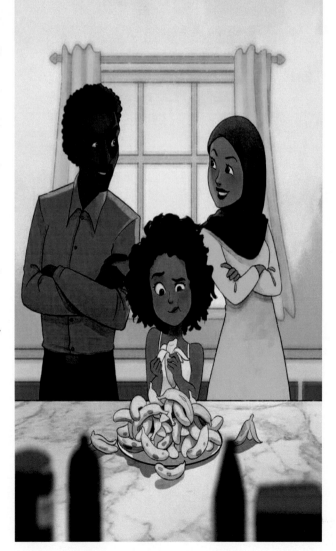